CW01509569

POEMS OF DEVOTION AND COMMOTION

This is the second book of poems by Iris Therese Smith Reid inspired by the experience of caring for a dementia sufferer. Her husband was diagnosed with dementia more than seven years ago, and since then Iris has chronicled the impact his illness has had on their life together. Her poems express what it really means when the connection between two people is held together by a great bond of devotion.

A selection of amusing verse ends the book in a lighter vein.

POEMS OF DEVOTION AND COMMOTION

Iris Therese Smith Reid

ARTHUR H. STOCKWELL LTD
Torrs Park, Ilfracombe, Devon, EX34 8BA
Established 1898
www.ahstockwell.co.uk

By the same author:

DEMENTIA POEMS

ISBN 978-0-7223-4722-5
Printed in Great Britain by
Arthur H. Stockwell Ltd
Torrs Park   Ilfracombe
Devon EX34 8BA

CONTENTS

Angel Carers	9
Stressful State	10
Damaged Mind	11
Make Him Better	12
Confusing Days	13
Not Allowed to Drive	14
Just a Little Prick	15
Jumping in the Night	16
Going Far Away	17
Lost and Found	18
Poems about You	19
Always Moaning	20
Get Out of Bed	21
Reading in the Dark	22
Trying to Communicate	23
Not to Blame	24
Cannot Walk	25
Don't Tell Me What to Do	26
Leave Me Be	27
Lucky Man	28
Travelling Anew	29
I Am Not Your Sister	30
Pointing Out the Way	31
I Am Off This Time	32
Living Life Again	33
Inspiration	34
Ticklish	35
Cannot Sleep	36
Pick Your Foot Up	37
Shared Memories	38
On a Diet	39
For Ever Take My Hand	40
One Moment of Your Time	41
Smiling Through	42
Thankful	43

My Heart Is Here with You   44
Will He Be Coming Home?   45
No Praise for Me   46
Father's Day   47
Mother's Day   48
He Should Be Shot   49
What Is the Score?   50
Walking Wounded, Walking Dead   51
I Cannot Find My Way   52
Call Out My Name   53
Close Call   54
Eye Test   55
Watching over You   56
You Can Lean on Me   57
Only Staying for One Day   58
One Day of My Own Time   59
Don't Go Against Me   60
Just Another Day   61
The Further You're Away   62
Mirror of Your Mind   63
Perfect Day   64
Wondrous Place   65
In the Darkness of the Night   66
Night and Day   67
Blind and Cannot See   68
A Right Storm   70
Last Shove   71
Summer Has Begun   72
You Mean the World to Me   73
They Are Our Children   74
Winter Has Begun   75
Precious Love   76
Unforgotten Love   77

AMUSING POEMS
Brothers Fighting   79
It Was My Brother   80

Looking Guilty   81
No Good Running   82
Grandad's Snoring   83
Broken Window   84
It Was Not My Brother   85
One Pound 50p.   86
Swearing   87
Bad Bath Time   88
Good Bath Time   89
Swearing Budgie   90
Toad in the Pond   91
My Friend My Teddy Bear   92
Mischievous Cat   93
Stalking Cat   94
Monkey Business   95
Pretty Robin   96
Bird-Feeding   97
Grey Squirrels   98
My Puppy   99
Little Hedgehog   100
Quacky   101
Lost Pup   102
Little Buzzing Bee   103
He Sat There Watching Me   104
Salvation Army   105
Dustbin Men   106
I Pulled the Big One   107
The One That Got Away   108
My First Dance   109
Going for a Haircut   110
What Is It You're Hiding?   111

ANGEL CARERS

All you angel carers,
I think you will agree
Caring for someone you love
Is hard as hard can be.

To watch them trying very hard
To do something for you –
Watching them struggling
Is a painful thing to do.

It takes up all our energy
To do the best we can –
Anything to make them feel
A proud, a better man.

There is nothing in this world
We would rather do;
We have often shed a tear
Doing all they needed us to.

All you angel carers,
I think you will agree
Caring for someone you love
Is hard as hard can be.

STRESSFUL STATE

I write these poems about you
While I am wide awake.
It gives me something else to do
To stop a stressful state.

You need a lot of care,
You need a lot of time –
What little I have left
I use to make a rhyme.

You don't do what you used to,
Although you always try.
All the things I do for you –
You always wonder why.

You always say thank you
To people who are kind.
And do what you need them to
Because you have a poorly mind.

I write these poems about you
While I am wide awake.
It gives me something else to do
To stop a stressful state.

DAMAGED MIND

You have got dementia –
You have a damaged mind.
I know you don't retain things –
It happens all the time.

Your mind it wanders everywhere –
There is no telling where you are.
You often want to catch a train
And travel way off far.

Every time that you are gone
I try to help, you see.
You have someone to lean on,
And that someone is me.

There is only so much I can do,
But to you I will be kind.
I will take good care of you –
I will never be unkind.

You have got dementia –
You have a damaged mind.
I know you don't retain things –
It happens all the time.

MAKE HIM BETTER

He's going to see the Doctor;
He's not feeling very well.
They will make him better.
They know – they can tell.

He has to keep a chart
Of every time he wees.
I know he does not like it –
He is not very pleased.

He knows that it's to help him –
They have told him so.
They will make him better,
But there's things they need to know.

The sooner they find out,
The sooner it will be.
They will put it right
So he's healthy, he will see.

He's going to see the Doctor;
He's not feeling very well.
They will make him better.
They know – they can tell.

CONFUSING DAYS

It's one of his confusing days –
He does not even know
If he wants to stay,
If he wants to go.

Some days are confusing days –
Which he has plenty of –
Sitting there staring,
Not even caring,
Not knowing where to go,
Not knowing who he is,
Not knowing what to say,
Not knowing where he's been,
Not knowing who he's seen.

Today is a confusing day –
He is not even there,
He has lost his way,
He is going nowhere.

It's one of his confusing days –
He does not even know
If he wants to stay,
If he wants to go.

NOT ALLOWED TO DRIVE

"Can I have the car keys?
I want to drive the car."
"Stop and listen to me:
You're not allowed to drive.

"You have not got a licence –
They took it away from you.
You are not able to drive it now –
You don't know what to do.

"I'm the one who drives it now.
I hope to help, you see.
You have got dementia –
You must leave it up to me.

"You don't know what you're doing.
You can never drive again
Because you don't know how –
Your illness is to blame."

"Can I have the car keys?
I want to drive the car."
"Stop and listen to me:
You're not allowed to drive."

JUST A LITTLE PRICK

We're going for our flu jabs –
We're having them today.
I really do believe in them –
They keep the flu away.

The needle I don't mind it;
But him, it makes him sick.
I tell him, "It won't hurt you!"
But he nearly has a fit.
I tell him, if he's bothered
To turn his head away –
"Don't watch the needle going in."
Then he won't feel a thing.
I tell him just to wait and see –
It's just a little prick.
I don't think he believes me –
He still says he feel sick.
He sits there with a brave face
When in comes the nurse.
He makes out he's a gentleman –
He tells me to go first.
When it comes to his turn –
He tells the nurse he's sick.
She tells him he won't feel it –
It's just a little prick.

We're going for our flu jabs –
We're having them today.
I really do believe in them –
They keep the flu away.

JUMPING IN THE NIGHT

I wish that you would lie straight –
You never lie just right.
You keep jumping up and down
Every minute of the night.

I'm not surprised you're jumping.
You know you're falling down
Because you're only half asleep –
You're lying half on the ground.

You're halfway in bed, you're halfway out,
Jumping through the night,
Falling and twitching,
Giving me a fright.

Your head is on the bed,
Your feet are on the ground –
I tried to pull your feet back in
To stop you falling down.

I wish that you would lie straight –
You never lie just right.
You keep jumping up and down
Every minute of the night.

GOING FAR AWAY

I'm going far away today –
I'm going 100 miles.
I wish you would not go away –
I wish you would stay awhile.

I know I cannot stop you –
You have to go sometimes.
There is nothing I can do
Because it's in your mind.

You always have to go away,
And you don't even know.
I wish that you would stay –
I wish you would not go.

Dementia takes you far away;
It takes you day by day.
No matter what we try to do
We never do get through to you.

I'm going far away today –
I'm going 100 miles.
I wish you would not go away –
I wish you would stay awhile.

LOST AND FOUND

Where are you?
Where have you gone?
I hope you haven't gone too far.
I know you're lost and alone,
Not knowing where you are.

I'm so worried I won't find you.
I've been looking everywhere –
I've been going round in circles,
Finding you nowhere.

Where would I be without you,
Not knowing you were there?
I wouldn't know what to do
If you were not here.

Thank goodness you are found –
Now I can start to breathe.
If you were not around
I know that I would grieve.

Where are you?
Where have you gone?
I hope you haven't gone too far.
I know you're lost and alone,
Not knowing where you are.

POEMS ABOUT YOU

I write these poems about you –
About things you're going through.
I have to try with all my might,
So I can keep awake at night,
To keep looking after you.

And so I do my writing
While looking after you.
It takes my mind off things,
Gives me something else to do.

We don't know what comes our way,
So sometimes I feel so blue.
So for my own sake
These poems I write about you.

I cannot leave you on your own –
There is no telling where you'd be.
I know you would be all alone
If you never did have me.

I write these poems about you –
About things you're going through.
I have to try with all my might,
So I can keep awake at night,
To keep looking after you.

ALWAYS MOANING

Why are you always moaning?
I wish you'd leave me be.
I wish you'd leave me well alone –
You always moan at me.

Why are you always moaning?
You do it all the time.
Everything is done for you –
Everything is always fine.

Why are you always moaning
And throwing things around?
You have everything you need –
Why throw things on the ground?

Why are you always moaning?
Is it something I have done?
Tell me what is wrong,
Then we can get along.

Why are you always moaning?
Can you find something else to do?
You're always giving me orders –
I'm for ever running after you.

Why are you always moaning?
I wish you'd leave me be.
I wish you'd leave me well alone –
You always moan at me.

GET OUT OF BED

Come on, get up, get out of bed.
Have you heard one word I've said?
I'm so fed up of telling you
There are lots of things we have to do.

Come on, get up, get out of bed –
Don't pretend you did not hear.
Come on, get up, come and see –
There is breakfast here for you and me.

Come on, get up, get out of bed –
Don't pretend that I'm not here.
I know that you're not sleeping –
I watched your eyes; I caught you peeping.

Come on, get up, get out of bed.
Have you heard one word I've said?
I'm so fed up of telling you
There are lots of things we have to do.

READING IN THE DARK

He sits in the dark
Reading his book.
What are you reading?
Can I have a look?

"You cannot read in the dark,"
I tell him with a smile.
"Yes, I can," he replies,
"I do it all the while."

"Let me help you see.
Let me put it right.
You haven't got X-ray eyes –
I will turn on the light."

"I can read it anywhere –
I don't need a light.
I often sit here reading,
Especially on a night."

"What is that you're telling me,
Saying you can see?
You haven't got that good a sight –
You cannot read without a light.

He sits in the dark
Reading his book.
What are you reading?
Can I have a look?

TRYING TO COMMUNICATE

He tries to communicate
While he goes on his way,
But all he ever has to say
It's a good day today.

I don't want to upset him –
He thinks he's doing well.
He thinks he is communicating
And I don't want to tell.

I always let him think
He has thought of what to say.
He will go along smiling –
It's a good day today.

It won't matter if it's snowing
Or teeming down with rain,
Gale-force winds blowing,
For all that's in his brain –
It's a good day today.

He tries to communicate
While he goes on his way,
But all he ever has to say
It's a good day today.

NOT TO BLAME

Every time I ask you
You keep telling me the same:
You had nothing to do with it,
You were not to blame.

There is only you and me here.
If it was not you, then who?
You tell me you were not there;
You tell me it's not you.

You said it wanted mending,
Telling me I did not know.
I told you it's not broken –
You know I told you so.

It's all right, do not worry,
I never used it anyway.
I was getting ready
To throw the thing away.

Every time I ask you
You keep telling me the same:
You had nothing to do with it,
You were not to blame.

CANNOT WALK

Don't tell me that you will not go
Because you cannot walk.
I don't mind pushing you around.
I think we need to talk.

I love to push you in your chair,
If that's what's on your mind –
Only because I care,
Not just because I'm kind.

I know you'd do the same for me
If it was me who could not walk.
Stop telling me to leave you be.
I think we need to talk.

For as long as possible,
I will always push you
Not because I don't want to
But because I do.

Don't tell me that you will not go
Because you cannot walk.
I don't mind pushing you around.
I think we need to talk.

DON'T TELL ME WHAT TO DO

Will you fetch my shoes for me
And take my plate with you,
Bring the paper for me to see
And take my cup out too?

Don't keep telling me what to do –
I'm not doing any more.
I know I do enough for you –
Of this I can be sure.

It's not that I don't want to –
I honestly don't mind.
While I'm doing everything for you,
To you I'm being unkind.

Because I am not helping you –
No exercise all the time.
So do the work you need to do
And I will just do mine.

Will you fetch my shoes for me
And take my plate with you,
Bring the paper for me to see
And take my cup out too?

LEAVE ME BE

Why do you pick on me
When I only do my best?
Why don't you leave me be,
When I never hardly rest?

I never have five minutes,
Though I know you won't agree.
I'm busy looking after you –
Why won't you leave me be?

When I hear you say
That I do nothing right,
Let me do my work today
So I don't work all night.

Why do you pick on me
When I've done nothing wrong?
Let me do my work in peace,
Then I'll soon be gone.

Why do you pick on me
When I only do my best?
Why don't you leave me be,
When I never hardly rest?

LUCKY MAN

Everybody cares for you,
Doing what they can.
Everybody is so kind –
You are a lucky man.

You don't know who you are,
You don't know what you do.
I am never far –
I'm watching over you.

I try to keep you safe.
In me you can confide.
I will keep you in your place.
I will be by your side.

Some days you'll go away –
With me it will be fine.
What has to be will be –
I can bide my time.

Everybody cares for you,
Doing what they can.
Everybody is so kind –
You are a lucky man.

TRAVELLING ANEW

He always lives a good life,
On holiday every day,
Travelling around the world,
But he never stays.

He travels everywhere –
Places I have never seen.
I would like to do the same
If only in my dream.

But it's not a dream for him,
He is actually there –
Not in his body, only in his mind,
But he won't need to care.

Oh to be on holiday,
No worries and no strife –
Nothing to do but laze around
Every day of your life.

Nobody to moan at you,
No work for you to do,
Just a happy scenic journey,
Travelling anew.

He always lives a good life,
On holiday every day,
Travelling around the world,
But he never stays.

I AM NOT YOUR SISTER

I am not your sister,
I am your loving wife.
I know you always say I am
And it cuts me like a knife.

I know you cannot help it,
What it is you say.
I know it's your dementia –
It will not go away.

I always try to put it right –
It's always been that way.
I try with all my might,
But dementia's there to stay.

Whatever you say or do,
I know that you do care.
You always think I'm not with you,
But I am always there.

I am not your sister,
I am your loving wife.
I know you always say I am
And it cuts me like a knife.

POINTING OUT THE WAY

He always takes his walking stick
When I push him in his chair,
Always pointing out the way
While going out somewhere.

When we go round corners
He shoots out his hand,
Whacking it left and right,
Not knowing where it lands.

When I'm going straight ahead
I really do see red.
He swings it front and back,
Whacking me upon my head.

If anyone is in the way,
They will get whacked too.
They will glare at him and say,
"Do you mind watching what you do!"

I have to take it off him
For he's a dangerous man.
He tries hanging on to it
For as long as he possibly can.

He always takes his walking stick
When I push him in his chair,
Always pointing out the way
While going out somewhere.

I AM OFF THIS TIME

For a long time now I've tried to tell you
What is on my mind,
But when I'm about to
I always feel unkind.

I have to say
I'm going away –
I am off this time.
I won't be gone
For very long –
You won't know I've gone.

I have to go into hospital
To have my knees both done.
Your daughter knows what to do –
She will take good care of you.

Don't you dare to play her up –
She will tell me if you do.
The both of you can wish me luck
And I'll be watching out for you.

For a long time now I've tried to tell you
What is on my mind,
But when I'm about to
I always feel unkind.

LIVING LIFE AGAIN

You live your life over.
You don't just think – you're there.
You are actually living it –
You are never here.

When you do relive your life
You have no worry and no fear.
You don't even have a wife;
You don't even care.

You're always going back in time,
Living in the past.
How long for? I never know
How long it will last.

Oh to live my life again –
Only the good times though!
Until then I'll dream in vain,
Until then I'll never know.

You are always here with me –
In body, not in mind.
I know you always go away
Nearly all the time.

You live your life over.
You don't just think – you're there.
You are actually living it –
You are never here.

INSPIRATION

I get my inspiration
From looking after you,
Listening to what you say,
Watching what you do.

I cannot leave you on your own –
With you I have to stay.
You would wander far from home;
You would leave and go away.

Every night I am alone
For you do not sleep.
I am sleeping on my own –
It's then that I do weep.

You never call me by my name –
It's then I shed a tear.
You never do remember me
Even though I'm always there.

I take you everywhere with me,
Even though you never know.
Everything I see, you see;
Everywhere I go, you go.

I get my inspiration
From looking after you,
Listening to what you say,
Watching what you do.

TICKLISH

Let me put your socks on –
Don't pull your feet away.
You're giggling
And wriggling,
Not wanting me to stay.

You cannot wear your shoes
Without your socks on,
So you have to let me try.
You won't let me touch your toes –
You're ticklish, that's why.

You have to let me help you –
You have to put them on.
You cannot do it on your own –
It does no good to want me gone.

It's no good you telling me
That I should leave you be.
Brave it – let me put them on
And the tickling will be gone.

Let me put your socks on –
Don't pull your feet away.
You're giggling
And wriggling,
Not wanting me to stay.

CANNOT SLEEP

I don't know why I cannot sleep –
I don't even get one wink.
I've even lain counting sheep,
But all I did was think.

Counting sheep won't work for me.
I'm tossing and turning,
Cussing and swearing –
My mind won't set me free.

That is why I cannot sleep –
I have too much on my mind.
For now my sleep will have to keep –
It's answers I must find.

I heard my old man snoring –
I was jealous as could be.
It should not be him sleeping –
That should have been me.

I had to get up out of bed
To think what it could be.
Then I knew why I could not sleep –
I had been drinking coffee.

I don't know why I cannot sleep –
I don't even get one wink.
I've even lain counting sheep,
But all I did was think.

PICK YOUR FOOT UP

Will you pick your foot up!
You keep dragging it along.
Everything that's on the floor
You drag with you once more.

I've told you many times before,
But you still will drag your foot.
The reason I keep telling you:
I don't want you tripping up.

I always have to walk with you
To stop you falling down.
I always show you what to do
Because you drag it on the ground.

When you walk, bend your knee –
Don't walk with a stiff leg.
If only you would listen to me
An improvement you will see.

I don't like to keep on at you,
But what else can I do?
I need to help you when I can
To make you be a better man.

Will you pick your foot up!
You keep dragging it along.
Everything that's on the floor
You drag with you once more.

SHARED MEMORIES

I share with him our memories,
I share with him our past.
I tell him one day at a time –
With him they do not last.

I tell him all about them –
Things we did and when.
He remembers for five minutes,
Then they're gone again.

I show him photos so he can see
Places where he went with me.
Places where we used to go
I can see he does not know.

I asked him what we used to do,
Where we went and with who,
Asking him what we had seen –
He does not know where he's been.

I show him his family –
I show him every day
Memories of him and them
That he's lost along his way.

I share with him our memories,
I share with him our past.
I tell him one day at a time –
With him they do not last.

ON A DIET

I have to put you on a diet,
Your nurse told me today.
When I push you in your chair
It takes my breath away.

You have got so heavy
I'm running out of puff.
I try so hard to push you,
But I have to give it up.

So now you're going to starve me
And I'll be skin and bone.
There won't be any fear of that –
It will take years to shift that fat.

Your nurse said you must diet
Before me or the chair break down.
It is going to be the chair,
That means you're going nowhere.

If it ends up being me,
Then where will you be?
I think you should give in –
I'm afraid the diet wins.

I have to put you on a diet,
Your nurse told me today.
When I push you in your chair
It takes my breath away.

FOR EVER TAKE MY HAND

Take my hand – I'll help you.
Swallow all your pride.
No matter what you say or do
I will stay by your side.
For ever take my hand.

Sometimes there is happiness,
Sometimes there is pain.
Accept my helping hand –
With you I will remain.
For ever take my hand.

When the sun is shining
We are happy; we are sad
When it starts raining –
We are miserable and sad.
For ever take my hand.

Come rain or shine,
No matter what,
I'm with you all the time.
We will always have a bond.
For ever take my hand.

Take my hand – I'll help you.
Swallow all your pride.
No matter what you say or do
I will stay by your side.
For ever take my hand.

ONE MOMENT OF YOUR TIME

Oh to have one moment –
One moment of your time.
Being with you for a while
Would make my life worthwhile.

Looking up at the stars
Twinkling oh so bright –
A feeling of contentment
On a darkened night.

No loneliness, no heartache
We would have to share,
No sadness, no heartbreak
We would have to bear.

Running on the sand,
Swimming in the sea,
Holding onto your hand,
You looking up at me.

One moment of peacefulness,
Tenderness and care,
One moment of togetherness
We could both share.

Oh to have one moment –
One moment of your time.
Being with you for a while
Would make my life worthwhile.

SMILING THROUGH

Put that smile back on your face
Just as it was before,
For there is no better place
That smile belongs for sure.

I see you going off to sleep
More throughout each day;
I see you're getting weak
As you go along your way.

All that I do ever see
Is you smiling back at me.
No matter how hard it is for you,
You still come smiling through.

You get yourself in such a muddle
Although you always try.
I don't like to see you struggle –
I feel like I could cry.

Put that smile back on your face
Just as it was before,
For there is no better place
That smile belongs for sure.

THANKFUL

You are always thankful,
Happy and kind.
You never let anything
Play upon your mind.

Everyone who comes your way
You always say good morning.
When they pass you by
You always say good day.

You are always happy
In everything you do.
You always have a smile –
Nothing worries you.

You never lose your kindness
As you go along your way.
You never lose your thankfulness,
Not even for a day.

You always give a handshake
And a moment of your time.
Everything you do and say
Makes it a better day.

You are always thankful,
Happy and kind.
You never let anything
Play upon your mind.

MY HEART IS HERE WITH YOU

It's no good you keep telling me
To go away and start anew.
I know where I want to be –
My heart is here with you.

I'm staying here – this is my life.
I don't want to start anew.
You're my husband, I'm your wife –
My heart is here with you.

I know you're feeling guilty
Because nothing can you do.
I know you blame yourself, but
My heart here with you.

There is no other place that I would rather be,
Nothing more I want to do.
I just need to make you see
My heart is here with you.

I will never go away,
No matter what you do.
I will always stay –
My heart is here with you.

It's no good you keep telling me
To go away and start anew.
I know where I want to be –
My heart is here with you.

WILL HE BE COMING HOME?

I know he has gone away,
I know he's gone again,
I know he cannot stay –
His illness is to blame.

Will he be gone one night?
Will he be gone one day?
He might be gone for ever –
He might even stay away.

One day he is here,
Next day he is gone.
I hope he won't stay there –
I hope he won't be long.

One day I do know,
Because I've been told so,
He more or less will stay,
So I take it day by day.

If he never does come back to me
I won't be on my own,
For he is here for me to see –
I won't be all alone.

I know he has gone away,
I know he's gone again,
I know he cannot stay –
His illness is to blame.

NO PRAISE FOR ME

Oh, he does so very well –
He looks so fit, you can tell.
After everything he's been through
He is so strong, I'm telling you.

Tell me about it, why don't you?
What about what I go through –
All the caring I have to do.
Washing and cleaning,
Bathing and feeding –
I'm run into the ground.
Hospitals, clinics,
Doctors and nurses,
Hearing him moaning,
Cursing and groaning –
There's me never making a sound.
I need a medal for what I go through
As if I've nothing else to do.
Him not knowing I'm even there –
Oh for someone to show they care!
I'm happy everyone praises he
If only there was praise for me,
The one who helps him stay alive,
The one who helps him to survive,
The one who's always there,
His one and only carer.

Oh, he does so very well –
He looks so fit, you can tell.
After everything he's been through
He is so strong, I'm telling you.

FATHER'S DAY

Today is very special
Because it's Father's Day.
The children are already there,
Showing him how much they care.

They brought him many gifts –
Lots of clothes to wear –
But his most precious gift of all
Was his children being there.

Today he is a happy man,
His children doing what they can
To be loving, to be kind,
Showing he is on their mind.

He loved all his presents,
He had lots of things to say,
He really did feel happy
On his Father's Day.

Today is very special
Because it's Father's Day.
The children are already there,
Showing him how much they care.

MOTHER'S DAY

Today is very special
Because it's Mother's Day.
All the children rang to say
They are on their way.

Bringing flowers with them,
Bringing all their fare,
They are very loving –
It's like a florist's shop in here.

While they are with me
I never need to fear.
They are very thoughtful,
Showing how they care.

It's not just Mother's Day, you see –
They are often here with me
For a chat, a cup of tea.
I'm so lucky they live near
Because sometimes I go there.

We are a close and loving family,
So joyful and so kind –
You could search around the world,
No better family you would find.

Today is very special
Because it's Mother's Day.
All the children rang to say
They are on their way.

HE SHOULD BE SHOT

It's a hospital visit for us today.
The times that we go there
We should take our bed with us –
We should just live here.

We have to see about his foot:
He cannot pick it up,
He cannot bend his knee,
So now he is as lame can be.

I tell him if he was a horse
By now he would be shot.
He would get the needle if it was up to me.
I tell him he's had his lot.

The nurse said to me she would like a word –
It was not as bad as she had feared.
She has done her very best;
Now he can go home to rest.

It's a hospital visit for us today.
The times that we go there
We should take our bed with us –
We should just live here.

WHAT IS THE SCORE?

"I've had a pain all night –
It comes and it goes.
Can you put it right?
I thought you need to know."

"Take a dose of this
To show what is amiss.
Tell me what's the score –
One to ten or more?"

"It started off at four
Then went away again,
Then it went to six, then more,
Now it feels like ten."

"Right, I'll call the Doctor
To see what's up with you."

"Can you wait for just a mo?
I must go to the loo.
That's it – I'm all done.
Now my pain has gone."

"So you just wanted the loo –
That is what was wrong with you."

"It was that medicine you gave me –
I know that now for sure.
That got to the bottom of it –
That did find the cure."

"I've had a pain all night –
It comes and it goes.
Can you put it right?
I thought you need to know."

WALKING WOUNDED, WALKING DEAD

When I look at you,
Knowing what you've been through,
Thoughts come in my head:
You are the walking wounded,
You are the walking dead.

I call him this, and him and me
Can see the funny side.
We both have afflictions that everyone can see
That we would soon hide.

I laugh at him, he laughs at me,
We break out in a grin.
If not, this place that we live in would be so sad
We would not want to live in.

Who knows what tomorrow brings?
Throw caution to the winds!
I make him happy when I can –
It makes him feel a better man.

When I look at you,
Knowing what you've been through,
Thoughts come in my head:
You are the walking wounded,
You are the walking dead.

I CANNOT FIND MY WAY

"Can you help me? I am lost –
I cannot find my way."
"Where is it that you want to go?"
"I don't know – I cannot say."

"Tell me where you live
And I will take you home."
"I don't remember where it is –
I wish I did not roam.

"I know I did not go too far –
I am not far away.
My wife told me not to go –
She told me not to stray.

"She said I would get lost
If I went out on my own.
She said I would be all alone
And not find my way home."

"Let us look inside your wallet –
Your ID might be in there
In cases where you tend to roam.
Yes it is – it is in here.
Now I can take you home."

"Can you help me? I am lost –
I cannot find my way."
"Where is it that you want to go?"
"I don't know – I cannot say."

CALL OUT MY NAME

You never do remember me –
You never remember my name.
Oh to hear you call me it –
To hear it once again!

My name will not come back to you
Whatever I say or do.
On your mind it does not stay –
It's gone clean away.

It's nearly half a year
Since you called out my name.
I am always waiting to hear,
But I wait in vain.

You don't even remember me,
You don't even know I'm here.
I don't know why I worry,
Because I know you care.

You never do remember me –
You never remember my name.
Oh to hear you call me it –
To hear it once again!

CLOSE CALL

I thought that was the end for you –
Six months not knowing if you would pull through,
Trips to hospital day and night,
Always praying you're all right.

Family staying by your bed,
Making sure that you were fed,
Making sure that you were fine,
Everybody being kind.

So many watching over you,
Fussing, not knowing what to do.
I won't forget when you awoke,
Making sure you did not choke.

Now you're home and doing fine,
Thanking all for being kind,
Knowing all that we did know,
Knowing it was touch and go.

I always knew you'd prove them wrong –
I always knew that you were strong.
I knew you'd come back home to me –
Back home to all your family.

I thought that was the end for you –
Six months not knowing if you would pull through,
Trips to hospital day and night,
Always praying you're all right.

EYE TEST

We're going for your eye test –
Come on, don't delay.
Come on, there's no time to rest –
We haven't got all day.

Your appointment is at three o'clock –
It's already quarter to three.
It's only just to check your eyes –
Don't worry, you will see.

Everything will be all right –
Your eyes look fine to me.
When nothing comes to light
They will leave you be.

I told you it would turn out fine.
You telling me you're going blind,
You telling me you cannot see,
Kicking up and frightening me!

You know I have enough to do
Without having to run after you,
Worrying about it on the way –
I told you that you were OK.

We're going for your eye test –
Come on, don't delay.
Come on, there's no time to rest –
We haven't got all day.

WATCHING OVER YOU

You should have popped your clogs by now,
The sickness you went through.
Someone's watching over you,
Watching what you do.

Different ailments day by day –
The pain you have endured.
Someone's looking after you,
The way you have been cured.

You are always happy,
Cheerful and carefree,
Getting on with your life,
Trying not to worry me.

Always quite contented
In everything you do,
Love and kindness spread around
All coming from you.

Believing all the good
In everyone you see –
Someone's watching out for you,
And that's including me.

You should have popped your clogs by now,
The sickness you went through.
Someone's watching over you,
Watching what you do.

YOU CAN LEAN ON ME

When you find it hard to come and go
I need to let you see –
I need to let you know
You can lean on me.

When you're crying and depressed
After trying your very best,
When you're down and full of fright
Because you cannot get things right
You can lean on me.

When you're upset and feeling low,
Feeling tired, wanting to go,
When you find it hard to breathe,
Feeling that you need to grieve,
You can lean on me.

When you think you're on your own,
A feelings of being all alone;
When you don't know what to do,
A feeling no one's there for you,
You can lean on me.

When you find it hard to come and go
I need to let you see –
I need to let you know
You can lean on me.

ONLY STAYING FOR ONE DAY

I know how you're feeling,
Wanting me to stay.
Don't worry, I'm not leaving –
You're only here for one day.

You know I would not leave you –
The things we have been through.
I'm not going away to stay –
You're only staying for one day.

You're having one day of therapy,
One day of exercise.
You will be with your friend
While I have other things to tend.

You always enjoy yourself,
You're never there to stay.
You have one day of freedom –
Don't throw it away.

When I come back for you
You tell me what to do –
To leave and go away.
You don't want me to stay.

I know how you're feeling,
Wanting me to stay.
Don't worry, I'm not leaving –
You're only here for one day.

ONE DAY OF MY OWN TIME

All I'm taking is one day –
One day that is all mine,
Just one day a week for me,
One day of my own time.

I will not feel guilty
You're now healthier than me.
I've helped you through your sickness,
I cannot help you with your mind.
All I'm taking is one day,
One day of my own time.

One day a week won't hurt you –
There are things I have to do.
To you I'm just your carer –
You don't even know I'm there.
All I'm taking is one day,
One day of my own time.

People will be there for you –
People who do care.
Now I'm looking after me;
I've looked after you a year.
All I'm taking is one day,
One day of my own time.

All I'm taking is one day –
One day that is all mine,
Just one day a week for me,
One day of my own time.

DON'T GO AGAINST ME

If you do what I ask you to,
The better for me and you,
The quicker it will be
If you don't go against me.

I do my best to dress you –
You make it hard for me to do.
Put your leg up, bend your knee,
Just don't go against me.

Your jumper is all twisted up,
Your trouser leg wrapped round your foot.
Make it easier for me to do,
Then I can put your socks on you.

You fastened up your buttons
In the wrong holes – such a shame.
Now I have to undo them
And fasten them again.

If you help me put your shoes on
It won't take us very long.
Pick your foot up, you will see,
Just don't go against me.

If you do what I ask you to,
The better for me and you,
The quicker it will be
If you don't go against me.

JUST ANOTHER DAY

I see that look upon your face –
You have gone away.
There is nothing I can do
That would help you stay,
So I have to tell myself it's just another day.

Once again you have to go,
Leaving me alone.
Now I feel this emptiness
Because I'm on my own
So I have to tell myself it's just another day.

There is no fun, no laughter,
No joy, nothing there,
Only this darkness,
Loneliness and fear,
So I have to tell myself it's just another day.

There is nothing I can say or do
Because it won't get through to you.
There is nothing I need to fear,
Because you're always there.
So I have to tell myself it's just another day.

I see that look upon your face –
You have gone away.
There is nothing I can do
That would help you stay,
So I have to tell myself it's just another day.

THE FURTHER YOU'RE AWAY

I want you to come home,
I want you to stay.
The further that you roam,
The further you're away.

You are neither here nor there,
You wander and you stray.
The further that you roam,
The further you're away.

We have lots of things to share,
Lots of things to say.
The further that you roam,
The further you're away.

You're always going somewhere,
Getting lost upon the way.
The further that you roam,
The further you're away.

You're busy going nowhere,
You're never there to stay.
The further that you roam,
The further you're away.

I want you to come home,
I want you to stay.
The further that you roam,
The further you're away.

MIRROR OF YOUR MIND

What is it you have found?
Love and happiness all around,
Loving friends all to find
Coming through the mirror of your mind.

Carers looking after you,
Respecting everything you do,
Everything all outlined
Coming through the mirror of your mind.

Songs and laughter in the air –
Lots of people really care.
So many, oh so kind,
Coming through the mirror of your mind.

Spreading joy everywhere,
So much so we all can share,
Everybody feeling fine
Coming through the mirror of your mind.

Singing, dancing, here and there,
Families all being here,
Some of yours, some of mine,
Coming through the mirror of your mind.

What is it you have found?
Love and happiness all around,
Loving friends all to find
Coming through the mirror of your mind.

PERFECT DAY

We sit staring at the sky,
Watching clouds go sailing by.
Never let it slip away –
This is just the perfect day.

It's so peaceful sitting here –
All our pains just disappear.
We could stay here all the day –
This is just the perfect day.

Then a plane goes flying by,
Leaving white trails in the sky.
The trails then fade, they do not stay –
This is just the perfect day.

Lots of geese are flying high,
Making patterns as they fly,
Then two rainbows in the sky
Make an arch then slip away –
This is just the perfect day.

We sit staring at the sky,
Watching clouds go sailing by.
Never let it slip away –
This is just the perfect day.

WONDROUS PLACE

Cliffs so high
Reach to the sky,
Sun so bright
Shining us a light,
Waterfalls running down
Into the lakes below –
There is no more wondrous place
I would wish to go.

Skies so blue
Like crystal ice,
Seas so green
Like emerald isle,
Mountains white
Laden with snow –
There is no more wondrous place
I would wish to go.

Enchanting forest
Filled with trees,
Desert dunes
With golden sand,
Green grass laid
Upon the land –
There is no more wondrous place
I would wish to go.

IN THE DARKNESS OF THE NIGHT

Silver shards spinning round
Like diamonds sparkling on the ground,
Dewdrops like dancing lights
In the darkness of the night.

A burning glow from fireflies
Lighting up the darkened skies,
A beautiful scenic sight
In the darkness of the night.

Foxes, cats out on the prowl
Diving on the waterfowl,
Howling wolves giving all a fright
In the darkness of the night.

Glow-worms glowing in the dark,
Glittering, shimmering like a spark,
Early song of a lark
In the darkness of the night.

Hooting owls from woods afar,
Crickets whistle all night long,
Nightingales sing a beautiful song
In the darkness of the night.

Silver shards spinning round
Like diamonds sparkling on the ground,
Dewdrops like dancing lights
In the darkness of the night.

NIGHT AND DAY

Daytime turning into night,
Lightness turning into dark,
Stars appear, twinkling bright,
Shining out a silver light.

A shooting star hurtles by,
Leaves sparkling lines in the sky,
The Milky Way in heavens far,
Leo and Venus, shining stars.

The Earth for ever spinning round,
Not a breath, not a sound.
The universe it has no end,
Eternity they do blend.

So many planets no one knows –
Life forever grows
Like day and night, like death and life
They all come and go.

Suddenly a shred of light
Breaks the darkness of the night,
Stars go out, they disappear
Leaving a different atmosphere.

A coloured sky, a morning dawn,
A yellow sun making warm,
Shining out a sheen of light,
Casting out the dark of night,
Lighting all along its way,
Night-time turning into day.

BLIND AND CANNOT SEE

Trust in me, I'll guide you.
Follow me, I'll see you through.
I am your faithful friend.
I know you're blind and cannot see –
Put your trust in me.

Stand up tall and be brave –
You don't have to feel afraid.
Have faith in me and you will see –
Put your trust in me.

I will never leave you on your own;
You will never be alone.
I will take you where you want to be –
Put your trust in me.

You're safe with me wherever you go;
Where you are I'll always know.
I know you cannot see –
Put your trust in me.

I will take good care of you –
To you I always will be true.
Stay close beside me –
Put your trust in me.

I'm here to show you what to do,
To take you along, to help you,
To guide a path along your way –
Put your trust in me.

Trust in me, I'll guide you.
Follow me, I'll see you through.
I am your faithful friend.
I know you're blind and cannot see –
Put your trust in me.

A RIGHT STORM

It started slowly coming down,
Wetting everything around,
Pattering on windowpane,
Slowly running down the drain.

The sun and bright sky disappear,
Then the hailstones they appear.
They're so big, they're so round,
Leaving large holes in the ground.

Heavens black they open wide,
Lightning and thunder side by side,
Wind whipping up a breeze,
Causing storms upon the seas.

Flooding land, uprooting trees,
Temperatures turn to freeze,
Howling gales blowing around
Hillsides, bridges falling down.

Then a calmness from up high,
Sun starts shining in the sky,
Quietness, not a sound,
Flowers peeping through the ground.

It started slowly coming down,
Wetting everything around,
Pattering on windowpane,
Slowly running down the drain.

LAST SHOVE

You told me you loved me for ever,
Saying we belong together.
I loved you until that fateful day
You told me to go along my way,
Saying you had another love
And you were giving me the shove.

My world just fell apart –
You just broke my heart.
You just threw our love away –
With me you did not want to stay.

Until one day you came back to me,
Hoping and begging I would see,
But I only had one thing to say:
My love for you had gone away.

It was my turn now to watch you go,
But I did not say I told you so.
I must admit I did feel glad,
Knowing your love had turned out bad.

I was happy with myself that day –
It was my turn now to have my say,
Telling you to go along your way,
Watching as you slinked away.
I told you I had another love
And I was giving you the shove.

SUMMER HAS BEGUN

Scenic buildings standing high,
Rivers running snake-like
Into the sea so blue
Where boats go sailing to,
Dolphins playing in the sea,
Doing tricks for you and me.
Yellow shining sun –
Summer has begun.

Fields and fields of golden corn,
Sheep are being shorn,
Lambs already born,
Little baby fawn.
Children play among the flowers –
Longer daytime hours.
Picking strawberries, having fun –
Summer has begun.

Tractors ploughing up the field,
Sowing in their seed,
Trying for their summer yield.
Haystacks for animals' feed,
Potato harvest being done
Before the setting of the sun.
Farmers on their daily run –
Summer has begun.

Fish are swimming in the sea –
Fishermen are catching some.
Sleeping seals for us to see,
Birds breaking out in song,
Country roads are winding,
Rock and mountain climbing,
Pheasants for the gun –
Summer has begun.

YOU MEAN THE WORLD TO ME

My eyes are open wide –
With you I feel alive.
I am not blind, my eyes can see –
You mean the world to me.

You are my shining light –
You guide me through each night.
Without you where would I be?
You mean the world to me.

I don't know what I'd do
If I never did have you.
Your love won't set me free –
You mean the world to me.

You are my brightest star –
My happiness is where you are.
You always fill my heart with glee –
You mean the world to me.

You are so full of love,
You are my little dove.
You are my destiny –
You mean the world to me.

My eyes are open wide –
With you I feel alive.
I am not blind, my eyes can see –
You mean the world to me.

THEY ARE OUR CHILDREN

Our grandchildren, our great-grandchildren,
Our daughters, our sons,
They are our children –
Their lives we begun.

We gave them life,
We gave them love –
They are our children,
Our flesh and blood.

They all know how much we care.
They all know how we do fear.
To them we always will be giving –
They are our reason to be living.

We will do anything to keep them near –
Our lives together we do share.
I myself I'd sacrifice –
For either one I'd give my life.

All of them we love them dear;
For them we always will be there.
We would never leave them ever –
We will always be together.

Our grandchildren, our great-grandchildren,
Our daughters, our sons,
They are our children –
Their lives we begun.

WINTER HAS BEGUN

Icy winds with frozen rain,
Jack Frost on windowpane,
Christmas trimmings being done,
Christmas songs being sung –
    Winter has begun.

Reindeer with their noses red,
Icicles hanging overhead,
Ponds frozen, full of ice,
People skating, having fun –
    Winter has begun.

Snow falling all around,
Spreading a blanket on the ground,
Sledging down the hillside,
Skiers on a mountain run –
    Winter has begun.

Children playing in the snow,
Little faces all aglow,
Building snowmen, having fun,
Throwing snowballs at their mum –
    Winter has begun.

Icy winds with frozen rain,
Jack Frost on windowpane,
Christmas trimmings being done,
Christmas songs being sung –
    Winter has begun.

PRECIOUS LOVE

A beam of light coming down,
Sunbeams dancing all around,
Then a pure-white turtle dove
Flying down from up above.
A white feather comes to land,
Falling straight into my hand –
A message from my precious love.

When time came for you to go
My world ended for me, I know.
I lost my precious love that day –
A gust of wind took you away.
I always thought that you would stay.
I stand there staring at the sky,
Asking myself, wondering why.
It's been a time since you were gone –
Thoughts of you take me along.
I see a bright shining star
Twinkling on me from afar.
I'm lost in memories all about you –
Your smile for ever coming through.
There are delicate petals in my hand –
There are your children, our special bond.

A beam of light coming down,
Sunbeams dancing all around,
Then a pure-white turtle dove
Flying down from up above.
A white feather comes to land,
Falling straight into my hand –
A message from my precious love.

UNFORGOTTEN LOVE

As waves come surging to the shore
You said you were mine for evermore.
Your love you trusted in my hand
When you put on my finger a golden wedding band.

You said we would always be together,
Forgetting no one lives for ever.
I took for granted your life with me –
I sailed along so willingly.

But how little did I know
That one day you would go,
Leaving memories of me and you
That will for ever see me through!

I know you loved me greatly, my eyes just did not see
Until the day you went from me.
It's then that I did know
Just how much I loved you so.

I think about you every day –
My heart, my love, with you will stay.
Your smile will never set me free –
There is no other love for me.

Your children, this I know:
How much you loved them so.
They love you just the same –
Their love for you will never change.

As waves come surging to the shore
You said you were mine for evermore.
Your love you trusted in my hand
When you put on my finger a golden wedding band.

AMUSING POEMS

BROTHERS FIGHTING

"Mum, I have to tell you,
But you won't be very pleased,
I smacked my brother in the face
Because he kicked me on my knees."

"OK, go and say you're sorry
For you know that he loves you;
And he can say he's sorry
For I know he loves you too."

"But, Mum, he kicked me first
Then said he would tell you.
Then I smacked him back
And said I would tell you too."

"So you both have hit each other,
Which none of you should do.
Brothers should not ever fight,
So shake hands, both of you.

"Now you both have made it up,
I'm very pleased to say.
Now no more fighting from the two of you –
Now go back out and play."

"Mum, I have to tell you,
But you won't be very pleased,
I smacked my brother in the face
Because he kicked me on my knees."

IT WAS MY BROTHER

"Nan, look what my brother's done:
He went and tripped me up.
Now my trousers are all torn
And my knee it is all cut."

"Nan, he is so fibbing –
I did not trip him up.
It was him, Nan, and I'm not kidding –
He jumped right on my foot."

"Nan, I am the wounded one –
Look, Nan, you will see.
I did nothing wrong,
But him he cut my knee."

"Nan, will you tell my mother?
She will be so mad at me.
Tell her it was my brother
And I'll show her my knee."

"You know what you two have to do:
Both own up to her.
I'm sticking up for none of you –
I think that only fair."

"Nan, look what my brother's done:
He went and tripped me up.
Now my trousers are all torn
And my knee it is all cut."

LOOKING GUILTY

"The both of you look guilty –
What is it you're not telling me?
What is it you're hiding
That you don't want me to see?

"If you do not own up
You know what I will do:
It will be the naughty step
For the both of you.

"From the look on your two faces
It was not very nice.
I think you'd better tell me
Or you both will pay the price."

"It was not me, Nanna;
It was my brother who
Drew a face on Grandad's baldy head
And said I'm not to tell you."

"Nanna, I admit it, I am easily led –
It was only a little face I drew,
And, Nanna, look and see.
If Grandad sends me up to bed
I will sneak my phone with me."

"The both of you look guilty –
What is it you're not telling me?
What is it you're hiding
That you don't want me to see?"

NO GOOD RUNNING

"Nanna, Grandad's been asleep
And we have had great fun.
Then we heard him waking,
So we both did run.

"We tied his shoes together
Then broke an egg on his bald head.
Then he started waking up –
That's when we both fled."

"You know what you two have to do:
Go back and untie his shoes,
Then wipe the egg back off his head.
If he awakes and catches you he will send you both to bed."

"But, Nanna, what if he is awake
And waiting for us to come?
We won't be able to get away –
We won't have chance to run.
He might smack us on our bum."

"That is the chance you have to take.
You both have had your fun –
You have to stay and face him,
It will do no good to run."

"Nanna, Grandad's been asleep
And we have had great fun.
Then we heard him waking,
So we both did run."

GRANDAD'S SNORING

"Look, Nan, Grandad's snoring,
His mouth is open wide.
It's opening and closing –
I think he's catching flies.

"Can I show my brother
That Grandad's catching flies?
Because he won't believe me,
He will say I'm telling lies."

"Go on, then, you can show him,
But don't you wake him up.
He has been awake all night
With his poorly, poorly foot."

"Nan, we have both seen him
And he is fast asleep,
So we took his wig off –
Come, look, come and peep."

"Put that wig back on his head
Before he wakes up and sees.
He will blame it all on me –
He won't be very pleased."

"Look, Nan, Grandad's snoring,
His mouth is open wide.
It's opening and closing –
I think he's catching flies."

BROKEN WINDOW

"Why did you break the window
Then say it was not you?
I told you always tell the truth,
It is the bravest honest thing to do.

"I said stay out of trouble –
I know that it was you;
You haven't got a double.
What you say to me has to be true."

"OK, I did not mean to do it,
I was only having fun.
The ball flew through the window –
It was then that I did run.

"Now that I have owned up,
Now what will you do?
Was it not the bravest
And most honest thing to tell you?"

"Right, don't play near the window
Next time you play a game,
Then it won't get broken
And you won't be to blame."

"Why did you break the window
Then say it was not you?
I told you always tell the truth,
It is the bravest honest thing to do."

IT WAS NOT MY BROTHER

"Who took all the chocolate
That I hid away?"
"It was not me, Nanna –
I've just been out to play.

"It must have been my brother.
He would not give me some –
I told him I would tell you.
He said that if I do he would blame it on to me
And whack me on my bum."

"Right, come with me and we will see
Which of you is to blame.
I will see who is fibbing me
And who should feel the shame.

"I hope you're telling me the truth
Because I soon will have the proof."
"I'm very sorry, Nanna, I have lied.
I knew that you'd soon see.
That is why I cried.
I came to tell you it was me.

"My brother he is not to blame
And I am well ashamed."
"You should never blame your brother
For wrong things that you do.
I am very pleased you owned up, though,
But it's the naughty step for you."

"Who took all the chocolate
That I hid away?"
"It was not me, Nanna –
I've just been out to play."

ONE POUND 50p.

"When I lost my tooth
The fairy left something for me,
But I wanted more, you see –
She only left me one pound 50p.

"When my brother lost his tooth
He got twice as much as me."
"He was not telling you the truth –
It was the same one pound 50p.

"Accept it and be glad – it does not work like that.
You should never ask for more.
Many children they get nothing
Because their families are so poor.

"And if that's the score –
You always wanting more –
I'll tell the fairy, she will see,
She will take back the one pound 50p."

"I am sorry, I am glad –
For other children I feel sad.
With you I do agree –
I'll take the one pound 50p."

"When I lost my tooth
The fairy left something for me,
But I wanted more, you see –
She only left me one pound 50p."

SWEARING

"My brother has been swearing –
I've told him once or twice.
My ears have both been burning –
I've told him he is not nice.

"I told him I would tell you;
He said he does not care,
But that if I do
I would get a big thick ear."

"Don't tell him you have told me,
Don't tell him that I know.
I will deal with him, you will see –
I will not let it go."

"But he said that if I tell you
He will say it is not true,
Saying you would see right through me,
Saying you would know."

"I've a feeling I've been had –
I think you're both as bad.
In future if I hear
Either one of you two swear
I will show the pair of you
Exactly what I'll do."

"My brother has been swearing –
I've told him once or twice.
My ears have both been burning –
I've told him he is not nice."

BAD BATH TIME

"You two have to have a bath
And I have work to do.
I don't want to hear one word
From either one of you."

"Mam, he's splashed soap in my eyes,
Now he's made me nearly blind
And he's made me cry –
That's not being kind.

"Mam, he nearly drowned me,
He poured water on my head
And he keeps on kicking my legs, see –
Now both my legs are dead."

"I was only trying to wash your hair –
You said I could help you.
Why do you keep shouting 'Mam'?
You know what she will do."

"Right, what is it that I said?
I know what I will do –
You two are going straight to bed,
I've had enough of you."

"You two have to have a bath
And I have work to do.
I don't want to hear one word
From either one of you."

GOOD BATH TIME

It's bath time for the two of you.
You can take a toy each too.
I don't want no falling out,
I want no excuse to shout.

Don't splash each other in the eyes –
I don't want you two to fight.
I don't want to hear no cries
While I am out of sight.

You can have five minutes playing
Then wash yourselves real nice.
I don't want to keep on saying –
I don't want to tell you twice.

I did not hear you crying out,
I did not have to shout.
You washed yourselves well too –
I'm very proud of both of you.

You two have been so good –
I'm pleased, I knew you would.
You can have your phones after tea
For being so good for me.

It's bath time for the two of you.
You can take a toy each too.
I don't want no falling out,
I want no excuse to shout.

SWEARING BUDGIE

We had a coloured budgie,
He was yellow, blue and green.
Billy was his name.
To us he was a scream.

When people came to see him
The air turned black and blue,
For that budgie he could swear
More than anyone could do.

Everybody laughed at him.
They all wanted to see
Was it the budgie swearing
Or was it really me?

Billy always flew and sat
On top of our front door,
Then he would start swearing
And the people shouted more.

Then he would start chittering
And getting really mad,
Pecking and pulling at anything,
Upset and looking sad.
So the people go away,
But they come back another day.

We had a coloured budgie,
He was yellow, blue and green.
Billy was his name.
To us he was a scream.

TOAD IN THE POND

There is a toad lives in our pond,
Croaking all the day.
It hops among the lilies
Then swims fast away.

It hopped upon a flower,
Causing it to sway,
Spinning it along,
Then hopped upon its way.

It tries to jump out of the pond,
But the sides are far too steep.
But it keeps on trying
Until it takes that one big leap.

It jumped so high it made it –
Its hard work was all done.
Then it hopped back in the pond,
Swimming down till it was gone.

There is a toad lives in our pond,
Croaking all the day.
It hops among the lilies
Then swims fast away.

MY FRIEND MY TEDDY BEAR

I have a friend my teddy bear,
Stays with me all the time.
I will keep him safe
For he is only mine.

He is always with me,
He is always there,
I know he's happy as can be –
He is my friend my teddy bear.

He always travels on my back,
I never leave him all alone.
He goes in my backpack,
He's never on his own.

When I go to bed at night
I take him there with me.
I never want to lose him,
So unhappy I would be.

Although he's rather shabby now
I still love him so.
I know he loves me too –
Everywhere I go he goes.

I have a friend my teddy bear,
Stays with me all the time.
I will keep him safe
For he is only mine.

MISCHIEVOUS CAT

I have a very mischievous cat –
She is into everything.
One day I found her sat
With a leg stuck in a tin.

She ran straight up a ladder
Thirty feet off the ground,
Then sat there meowing
Because she could not get back down.

Her head was in the goldfish bowl,
Sticking out of it her legs;
I put sunglasses on her eyes
And she sits up and begs.

I made a little hammock
So she could have a swing.
It just makes her go to sleep
So then I can sleep in.

I have a very mischievous cat –
She is into everything.
One day I found her sat
With a leg stuck in a tin.

STALKING CAT

There is a cat comes in our garden
And it tickles me –
It sits there waiting patiently,
Stalking any birds it sees.

It creeps along the tree,
Hoping the birds don't see;
Then suddenly it pounces,
Then the birds all flee.

The birds are very crafty:
They wait for it to run,
Then they fly down on it,
Pecking it hard upon its bum.

It will start meowing
As it sneaks away,
Licking at its wounds
As it goes on its way.

Slowly glancing back,
Then running fast away,
Hoping they are there
When it comes back another day.

There is a cat comes in our garden
And it tickles me –
It sits there waiting patiently,
Stalking any birds it sees.

MONKEY BUSINESS

I have a cheeky monkey,
Cammo is his name.
He is so very cheeky,
Always playing games.

One day he jumped on someone's head,
Pulling out his hair,
Then stuck a finger up his nose –
I pretended I was not there.

Another day, another time,
He did a wee on someone's knee.
I said he was not mine;
I said he was not with me.

It was very late one night,
Cammo was swinging on the light.
When it came crashing down
I was so shocked I ran and hid, trying not to make a sound,

Thinking, 'That's it – I will get done,
Cammo will be gone for sure.'
When I got caught I shouted out,
Disowning him once more.

If I told Mother I was easily led
I hoped it would all turn out fine.
She confined Cammo to his bed,
Then confined me to mine.

I have a cheeky monkey,
Cammo is his name.
He is so very cheeky,
Always playing games.

PRETTY ROBIN

There is a pretty robin
Comes in our garden every day,
Giving us so much joy,
Watching it at play.

It hops among the flowers,
Eating up the seeds,
Dives into the lily pond
Then dries its feathers in the breeze.

Flies among the heather,
Cooling itself down,
Dives upon a worm,
Pulling it out the ground.

Then all the other birds
All come out to play,
It knocks them off their perches
Then it flies away.

Flying onto the bird 'seeder',
Spinning it around,
It goes round in circles
Until it ends up on the ground.

There is a pretty robin
Comes in our garden every day,
Giving us so much joy,
Watching it at play.

BIRD-FEEDING

I love to see the coloured birds –
I feed them every day.
As for crows and pigeons,
I wish they would go away.

I have to stay under cover
From the crows when they do hover,
Because they poo upon my head.
So they get no seed from me,
Because they make me flee.

The pigeons go too far,
Because they poo upon my car.
I have not fed them yet,
Because I'd sooner wring their neck.

The robins are so nice,
So I do feed them twice.
The doves are full of love,
So I feed them with kid gloves.

The little jenny wren,
I feed her there and then.
The finches I feed more –
Their colours I go for.

I love to see the coloured birds –
I feed them every day.
As for crows and pigeons,
I wish they would go away.

GREY SQUIRRELS

There are two grey squirrels playing in our trees,
Having so much fun,
Doing as they please
While both on the run.

Running up and down,
Then hiding well behind,
Running from each other
Then peeping all around.

Jumping up from off the ground
Then running up the tree,
Dodging round and round
So the other one won't see.

Then coming to a standstill
And lying flat upon the tree,
Outstretching all their feet,
Playing dead for all to see.

They then stop playing dead,
Start pulling each other by the head,
Dragging each other along
Until they both have gone.

There are two grey squirrels playing in our trees,
Having so much fun,
Doing as they please
While both on the run.

MY PUPPY

I have a little puppy,
I take him to the park.
When he spots another pup
He always stops to bark.

I always keep a lead on him –
I won't let him run away.
Because he's always trying to
I keep telling him to stay.

If he does a whoopsie,
I stop and pick it up.
I put my rubber gloves on
Because he is my little pup.

I keep him nice and clean,
I wash him every week.
I comb his fur to make him gleam,
I keep him tidy, I keep him neat.

I need everyone to know,
I need everyone to see
That I love him so,
And I know that he loves me.

I have a little puppy,
I take him to the park.
When he spots another pup
He always stops to bark.

LITTLE HEDGEHOG

"Look at that little hedgehog –
I'll go pick it up."
"I would not do that if I was you.
If you do, I wish you luck.

"It will stick its spines into you
Then roll into a ball,
Then I know what you will do:
You will let it fall."

"If I'm very gentle,
It won't do me any harm.
I can softly cuddle it,
I can keep it nice and warm.

"I know what we both can do:
I'll give it something to eat.
Then when it falls fast asleep
You can cuddle it too."

"I think I'll pass on that.
I think you are a silly bat.
There are some things I just will not do,
So I will leave it up to you."

"Look at that little hedgehog –
I'll go pick it up."
"I would not do that if I was you.
If you do, I wish you luck."

QUACKY

I have a baby duckling –
He stays in our pond.
He takes the bread out of my hand,
Of him I'm rather fond.

The only trouble is
He quacks away all night;
Then I cannot sleep,
So I have to put it right.

I've already thought of something
So I can sleep at night:
I will put my earplugs in –
That will put it right.

I have called him Quacky
Because I like that name.
My friends say I am whacky
And I should feel ashamed.

But I just ignore them –
I don't feel the shame,
For he is my baby duckling
And I love his name.

I have a baby duckling –
He stays in our pond.
He takes the bread out of my hand,
Of him I'm rather fond.

LOST PUP

I have lost my pup today,
I think he's wandered far away.
I only have one thing to say:
Come back home to stay.

I hope you were not led away;
I hope you're only out to play.
You're my pup, come back this way –
Come back home to stay.

I hope you're coming home today;
I hope you haven't gone astray.
I've been waiting all the day –
Come back home to stay.

I've searched every highway,
I've searched every low way,
I've been searching all the day –
Come back home to stay.

I have left you out a tray –
All your favourites on display.
I hope that you are on your way –
Come back home to stay.

I have lost my pup today,
I think he's wandered far away.
I only have one thing to say:
Come back home to stay.

LITTLE BUZZING BEE

We sat together in the park.
A bird was singing like a lark
When suddenly he said to me,
"What is that upon your knee?"
I looked down – what did I see?
It was a little buzzing bee.

He said to me, "Just keep calm.
That little bee will do no harm.
It will not stay there very long –
If you stay still it will be gone."

I tried my best with all my might
Not to give that little bee a fright.
I said, "Don't sting me, little bee.
I'm more afraid of you than you're afraid of me."

It looked at me as if to say,
"Don't worry, I am on my way."
With that it upped and flew away –
I was so happy it did not stay.

We sat together in the park.
A bird was singing like a lark
When suddenly he said to me,
"What is that upon your knee?"
I looked down – what did I see?
It was a little buzzing bee.

HE SAT THERE WATCHING ME

I was mowing the lawn for him to see
When suddenly I saw a bee –
It was heading straight for me,
Landing down upon my knee.
Him, he sat there watching me.

It was then that I did flee,
Thrashing wildly at that bee.
I was frightened as could be –
Did he not hear my mournful plea?
No, he just sat watching me.

He started laughing out with glee
At me trying my best to flee,
The bee still flying after me.
I was as angry as could be;
He sat laughing, watching me.

The bee then flew away from me,
I was happy as could be.
That was very hard for me,
Running frantically from that bee
While he just sat there watching me.

"I would be better off without thee!
You saw that bee trying to sting me.
You could have helped me from that bee –
That's the end of you and me.
How could you sit there watching me?"

I was mowing the lawn for him to see
When suddenly I saw a bee –
It was heading straight for me,
Landing down upon my knee.
Him, he sat there watching me.

SALVATION ARMY

The Salvation Army came down our street
Singing their hymns,
Rattling their tins
On Sunday once a week.

When we saw them,
My friends and me,
We picked on them
Relentlessly.

Until one day my mother's eyes
Looking at me in surprise –
From that look I could see
Punishment on the way for me.

It would do us no good to run away,
I knew then that we had to stay.
That was the end of all our fun,
Ending sooner than it begun.

The Salvation Army ignored our pleas,
We had to help them with their fees,
We had to pay for our sins:
We had to rattle all their tins.

The Salvation Army came down our street
Singing their hymns,
Rattling their tins
On Sunday once a week.

DUSTBIN MEN

What is all that noise?
What are all those sounds?
Oh, it's just the dustbin men;
They are on their rounds.

They won't be wanting my bin,
Because I've put nothing in.
There is nothing here to empty.
Tell that to the dustbin men;
Tell them there's nothing in.

What is that we heard you say?
Dustbin men, indeed!
That word to us is such a sin –
Refuse collectors,
Waste distributors,
Madam, if you don't mind!
But I'm sure there is rubbish for us to find –
We could put you in our bin.

What is all that noise?
What are all those sounds?
Oh, it's just the dustbin men;
They are on their rounds.

I PULLED THE BIG ONE

I've been sat here fishing,
I've been here all the day.
If I catch the big one,
With me it will stay.

I just had a fright –
I think I've got a bite.
My float is going round,
My rod is going up and down.

It feels like a big one
I've been reeling in a while.
I've got my net ready,
On my face I have a smile.

At last I've caught the big one –
I felt so big and strong.
When I saw it I felt sorry;
I thought that this is wrong.

I picked up my big one,
Thinking it's a sin.
I weighed it, I measured it,
Then put the fish back in.

I had pulled the big one –
With me it did not stay.
I stood there watching it
As it swam away.

THE ONE THAT GOT AWAY

I went fishing on my holiday,
I was fishing half the night.
Suddenly my rod jumped –
I had got a bite.

I spent a long time reeling in,
It put up a frantic fight.
It dragged me to the ground,
Spinning me around.

I saw it before I hit the floor –
What a sight to see!
It was the biggest barracuda
Looking back at me.

It was dragging me, catching me,
Pulling me towards the sea.
It very nearly pulled me in –
I was not going to let it win.

I got my foot against a rock –
It's there that I did stay,
Doing my best to stand my ground,
Getting the line securing it around.
It pulled the lot out of my hand
And then swam fast away.

I had tried all night to pull that fish out.
It had tried all night to pull me in.
Neither of us wanted to quit –
In the end the fish did win.

MY FIRST DANCE

I'm learning how to dance today –
I really need to learn.
I always have to walk away,
But I would like a turn.

I will try my very best
Now I have got a chance,
For I will not rest
Until I've had my first dance.

At last I have beaten it –
I know I really tried.
I know now I don't have to sit –
I can show off my stride.

Now I have to try and be
So calm so they don't see.
I cannot show I'm nervous –
They are all watching me.

I know I'm not an expert,
But I know that I did well.
In fact, I did do great;
In fact, my head did swell.

I'm learning how to dance today –
I really need to learn.
I always have to walk away,
But I would like a turn.

GOING FOR A HAIRCUT

I'm going for a haircut,
I want short back and sides.
I have a bald spot on the top,
But my hat will hide that lot.

I should buy a toupee,
So my wife has always said.
Give me back what you cut off –
She can stick it on top of my head.

It makes me look much younger,
My hairdresser she tells me,
But when I look in the mirror
I'm afraid I do not see.

I think she is just kidding me,
But I admit it does look nice.
That alone is worth a fee;
That alone is worth the price.

But I do look rather handsome
And I do look rather grand.
My wife tells me I'm living
In cloud cuckoo land.

I'm going for a haircut,
I want short back and sides.
I have a bald spot on the top,
But my hat will hide that lot.

WHAT IS IT YOU'RE HIDING?

He has something on his mind
And he's not telling me.
I am feeling well annoyed –
Whatever can it be?

I see he's hiding something
He does not want to share,
Leaving me to think what can it be?
Knowing that I care.

We tell each other everything,
So what's he got to hide.
We always work it out
Standing side by side.

I think I know what he's hiding –
I hope it is a ring.
That is why he won't say why;
That is why he's being sly.

OK, I will tell you:
On my walk I fell and tripped.
I did not know what to do
Because my trousers were all ripped.

All that fuss, all that taboo –
I'm so upset and mad at you.
You do get on my wick.
I will sew them up for you –
You are a silly twit!

He has something on his mind
And he's not telling me.
I am feeling well annoyed –
Whatever can it be?